The Fat to Fit Meltdown Manual

Create Weapons of Mass Reduction in Your Community

Carole Carson

Hound Press

Hound Press
P.O. Box 2328, Nevada City, CA 95959
Tel: (530) 478-5709 Fax: (530) 478-1108 www.HoundPress.com

Ordering Information

Quantity sales. Special discounts are available on quantity purchases by corporations, associations, and others. For details, contact the "Special Sales Department" at the Hound Press address above.

Individual sales. Hound Press publications are available through most bookstores. They can also be ordered directly from Hound Press: Tel: (866) 337-7836; Fax: (530) 478-1108, www.HoundPress.com.

Orders by U.S. trade bookstores and wholesalers. Please contact Independent Publishers Group, 814 North Franklin Street, Chicago, IL 60610 Tel: (312) 337-0747; Fax (312) 337-5983.

Printed in the United States of America

Interior design by Sue Knopf, Graffolio

Acknowledgments

Elisa Parker made significant conceptual and editorial contributions in the creation of this manual. Sue Knopf, Graffiolo, designed the interior.

ISBN: 978-0-9766030-5-4

First Edition
13 12 11 10 09 08 10 9 8 7 6 5 4 3 2 1

Disclaimer

This manual provides information on how to encourage changes in lifestyle resulting in greater fitness for members of your community. It is sold with the understanding that neither the publisher nor the author is engaged in rendering medical, psychiatric, or other professional services. If expert assistance is required, the services of a competent professional need to be sought.

The purpose of this manual is to encourage individuals and communities to become more fit. The author and Hound Press, a division of Baskerville Enterprises, LLC, shall have neither liability nor responsibility to any person or entity with respect to any damage caused, or alleged to have been caused, directly or indirectly, by information provided in this manual. If you do not wish to be bound by the above, you may return the manual within thirty days of purchase, together with proof of purchase, to the publisher for a full refund.

Contents

another, even as we support our teammates and, through our larger effort, support healthful changes in everyone around us.

Whichever perspective you choose, the purpose remains the same—to help people make friends, have fun, get fit, and lose weight together!

To that end, I've created this manual to provide information and instruction on how to create your own unique Community Meltdown to promote more healthful living. The concepts can be used to create an event for one thousand or as many as ten thousand participants. The choice is yours to make. How big is your vision?

The Community Meltdown encompasses efforts by individuals and teams to exercise and eat more healthfully throughout the day, whatever the setting—whether at home, work, or school. For purposes of clarity, I use the word "event" to describe the Community Meltdown in its entirety. The formal program consists of a series of structured weekly public meetings, which I refer to as "sessions." The jobs of the core team members, whom I refer to as "event organizers," are summarized in the body of the manual; detailed job descriptions are included in the appendix. I've also included forms in the appendix that I hope you will find helpful in the creation and execution of your Community Meltdown.

This manual is a living, growing, and incomplete document. I've left space for notes at the end of each section so you can jot reminders to yourself and add your own ideas. At the conclusion of your event, I'll want to get your suggestions on how the manual could be made more useful. Each event builds on prior events. As our experience grows, our advice and assistance can become more targeted so that even more communities can realize their fitness goals.

Writing a manual is not something that I'd normally consider "fun," yet this project was a labor of love. Throughout the work of writing and editing, I delighted in the knowledge that readers such as you would make good use of the material. Although I may never meet the people who will ultimately use this material, I do know for certain that we share a common passion for building stronger, healthier communities. Let the fun begin!

Overview

There are many wonderful things that will never be done if you do not do them.
—CHARLES D. GILL

Anyone who looks around can see that the majority of people in the United States are overweight. Approximately half of those overweight people are considered obese. That is, they are more than 20 percent over their ideal weight. In the last twenty years, the rate of morbid obesity (over one hundred pounds overweight) has increased from one in two hundred to one in fifty people (National Center for Health Statistics, Centers for Disease Control and Prevention).

Even more worrisome, childhood obesity is increasing at an alarming rate. Since 1980, the proportion of overweight children ages six to eleven has doubled, and the number of overweight adolescents has tripled (Centers for Disease Control and Prevention, "Prevalence of Overweight among U.S. Children and Adolescents"). This may be the first generation of children who will not live as long or as healthfully as their parents.

Obesity isn't contained within our country's borders either. It has spread worldwide. The World Health Organization, which coined the word "globesity," considers this public health issue to be as critical an issue as starvation and malnutrition. Setting aside the personal inconvenience and emotional distress of being overweight, the medical and financial consequences are staggering.

The solution is as obvious as the problem. We need to take action. We must tackle the challenge of obesity together. By promoting exercise and healthful eating, we raise the awareness of everyone—young and old, professional and volunteer, teacher and student.

Principles of the Community Meltdown Program: FIT

In recommending this solution, we underscore several key values whose first letters spell *FIT*:

F = Fun: Do you remember as a child how much fun it was to play outdoors with your friends? How you took your ability to move and run for granted? Even as adults, few joys compare with the hours we spend playing with our family and friends. That's the foundation on which the Community Meltdown is built. Having fun together, we can tackle our private and previously embarrassing concerns about being overweight and underexercised.

We believe that exercise is fun and recreational, a form of adult play. We encourage participants to be imaginative about exercising, whether it's walking llamas or waltzing. We also encourage participants to enjoy eating in new ways, experimenting with different foods, and preparing them in ways that promote health. And we also promote the fun of learning, of being open to new ideas. There is no destination, only the pleasure and joy of a journey with friends and family.

I = Individualized: One size doesn't fit all—we encourage exploration of what works for each person. Our program has no doctrine. No single diet or exercise is recommended. We encourage each person to find a lifestyle that can be joyfully sustained. We acknowledge that sometimes we fall off track. But we believe that eventually these dysfunctional impulses can be overridden by a stronger desire to lose weight and get fit.

To help individuals discover their unique needs and patterns, we recommend keeping a food journal. We also recommend daily exercise. We discourage dieting because it is not sustainable. We don't endorse any commercial products. Participants are encouraged to see a doctor before beginning an exercise regimen.

T = Teamwork Together: We believe that ordinary people working together can accomplish extraordinary things. Being part of a team makes us more accountable than we would be working alone. Sharing problems lightens the load and doubles the joy when our goal is reached.

When we publicly admit our need to get fit, we remove the option of quitting or regressing. We achieve more when we are part of a network of committed participants. Competition between teams is playful. A win-win outcome for everyone occurs when one team succeeds and shows another team how to succeed too.

Principles of Creating a Community Meltdown Event: FIT

The same three concepts apply to the creation and management of a Community Meltdown:

F = Fun: Creating this event needs to be fun for event organizers. At some point during the press of tasks you must handle to produce your Community Meltdown, you may forget to have fun. Remembering this concept will restore your perspective and help you stay in touch with your vision.

I = Individualized: Every community is unique. To achieve maximum impact, each program must be relevant, timely, and tailored to the individual community.

T = Teamwork Together: Everyone needs to participate, including medical experts, media, fitness club owners, businesses, employers, government officials, religious leaders, employees, and family members.

With these three concepts in place, you are now ready to take the first step in creating your own fun-filled, uniquely original Community Meltdown.

1. Turn Ideas into Action

It's kind of fun to do the impossible.
—WALT DISNEY

Most of us know the changes we need to make to lead a more healthful lifestyle. Many of us struggle to make those changes. When we experience repeated failures, some of us give up. The more persistent may try the latest fad diet.

Over time, though, we have become increasingly aware that if we are to achieve meaningful, sustainable changes in how we live, we must do it together. We must take public our private concerns about weight and lack of fitness. Only in that way can we give and receive the mutual support we need to succeed.

Although one person cannot make a commitment for an entire community, one person can decide to step forward and provide leadership in promoting healthier lifestyles. This person's public decision will allow us to focus our efforts and work together to bring about change. The leader should have not only a vision of a healthy community but also the skills to translate that vision into a practical reality. This person becomes a catalyst for change. When this person steps forward, we will be able to move collectively toward our community goal of more healthful lifestyles.

A popular, well-known person with a strong personality is the ideal catalyst for a Community Meltdown. As the event's spokesperson, he or she will invite others to join in taking action. Ideally, this is a person who has no financial interest in the outcome of the event and whose own lifestyle is an example of a commitment to fitness.

To maintain the integrity of the program, the spokesperson must model the behaviors that are encouraged in others. That doesn't mean the spokesperson must have achieved perfect fitness—he or she may be working toward a goal—but the spokesperson needs to be publicly committed to personal fitness.

The spokesperson is likely to make the decision to create a Community Meltdown without knowing how it will be organized, where resources will come from, or what kind of results will be achieved. The first critical step is simply to decide to begin.

Notes

2. Create Magic and Power

Life is a great big canvas and you should throw all the paint you can on it.
—DANNY KAYE

One of the first tasks of the spokesperson is to pick a clever and meaningful name for the event—relevant to your specific community. In our case, it was the "Nevada County Meltdown." A phrase or tagline needs to be added to the name. We used "Ordinary People Doing Extraordinary Things."

A successful Community Meltdown requires the help and participation of all segments of the community. After selecting the name, the spokesperson needs to issue a public invitation and challenge in print, on radio, on television, and through e-mail networks, thereby seeking pledges of support from all quarters. The spokesperson needs to look throughout the community for people, organizations, and businesses that can provide assistance.

Besides making public statements of support, diverse community entities and groups need to be enrolled in promoting the program through their own unique networks. Examples of groups and networks to be targeted for endorsement and active promotion of the Community Meltdown are given here. Because each community is unique, the targeted groups will be unique too. While lining up widespread support, the spokesperson can also be canvassing organizations as part of a second effort to recruit core team members for the jobs outlined in the next chapter.

Funding: The spokesperson needs to line up sponsors to cover the expenses of the Community Meltdown. Much of the cost of the event may be donated. Expenses might include those for facility rental, printed materials, phone, office, promotional materials, prizes, and advertisements.

Facilities: The spokesperson needs to consider available venues, such as auditoriums, sports stadiums, and other locations that are large enough to hold all the participants.

Media: The spokesperson needs to cultivate relationships with the various media in the community. All media must be engaged, including newspapers, radio, television, e-mail networks, and blogs.

Volunteers: The spokesperson needs to begin identifying the networks of volunteers that could contribute to a Community Meltdown.

Fitness community: The spokesperson needs to begin identifying leaders in fitness centers and other fitness professionals who are eager to encourage healthier lifestyles. The spokesperson can ask fitness club owners to donate passes to participants or arrange special classes for participants. All groups promoting fitness can be encouraged to give visible support by disseminating information through each of their networks.

Medical community: The spokesperson needs to contact leaders in the medical community. This network may include hospitals, physicians, physical therapists, clinics, HMOs, dentists, and other practitioners who are already working to improve the health of their patients.

Political community: The spokesperson needs to contact elected officials for support. Government endorsements can be in the form of proclamations or public statements of support at the state, county, city, and regional levels from the governor, county supervisors, mayors, city council members, state assemblypersons, and others. (See the sample proclamation in the appendix.)

Business community and public and private institutions: The spokesperson needs to ask major employers, especially if the employers are insurance and healthcare providers, to become stakeholders in promoting the Community Meltdown. Employers need to be asked to donate funds for expenses and prizes, form teams, and offer in-house services and programs in support of employee fitness. Categories of employers may include universities, colleges, schools, newspapers, radio stations, banks, real estate developers, and other major institutions, both public and private.

Service groups and community organizations: The spokesperson needs to involve service groups (such as United Way, Rotary, Soroptimist, the Elks, and Shriners) as well as churches, synagogues, and other religious organizations. These organizations need to be asked to promote the

Community Meltdown through their membership and e-mail networks. They can also form teams to participate. In addition, the spokesperson should encourage other groups that routinely have exposure to the public in a variety of settings—historical societies, museums, libraries, theater groups—to spread information about the Community Meltdown.

Entertainers, restaurateurs, and theater owners: The spokesperson needs to invite restaurateurs, in particular, to participate by offering on their menus healthy items featuring the Community Meltdown name. Movie theater owners and performers at entertainment venues can make announcements about the Community Meltdown before their programs begin.

Administrators and professional advisers: The spokesperson also needs to begin locating volunteers to help with phone calls, office work, and other administrative tasks. In addition, the spokesperson needs to find professional personnel who will donate their time in their field of expertise, be it medical, legal, or media relations.

To garner community support from these diverse groups, the spokesperson needs an effective team of event organizers, a core group that divides up the work and gets it done with minimal supervision. The next section lists those players and outlines their tasks. These core team members, most of whom will be volunteers, will likely share a passion for fitness. Working together creatively and with a sense of joy, they have the privilege of engineering an uplifting, memorable experience for their entire community.

Notes

3. Assemble the Core Team

Don't look at your feet to see if you are doing it right. Just dance.

—KOBI YAMADA

The spokesperson needs to recruit ten to twelve people to form a core team to organize and present the event. These people need to represent a cross section of the community, for example, leaders from the medical community, private businesses, government, and educational organizations. They also need to share a passion for fitness. This nucleus group will be asked to make and implement decisions with a high level of coordination and a minimal level of supervision.

Although these individuals may be volunteers, the work they do must be executed to the highest professional standards. The jobs described below can be assigned to individuals, or one person may wear several hats.

Beginning with the spokesperson, the responsibilities of the core team members are summarized below. See the appendix for detailed job descriptions that include a list of the key tasks assigned to each core team member.

Spokesperson: As noted earlier, the spokesperson serves as a catalyst for change in the community. To be effective, the spokesperson needs to have access to networks and associations across a broad spectrum of the community. He or she needs to be articulate, persuasive, and credible. This person represents the "face" of the Community Meltdown in the community and to the media. The spokesperson does not need to be perfectly fit but does need to demonstrate by intent and actions a commitment to living healthfully.

Chief executive officer: The second most critical role is that of chief executive officer (CEO). The spokesperson may elect to perform this role or assign the day-to-day responsibility for orchestrating and managing the event to a CEO. In either case, the highly skilled execution of the CEO's tasks is critical to the success of the Community Meltdown. The CEO has the difficult task of taking a vision—the idea of promoting community fitness—and translating it into a reality.

Media adviser: The media adviser's role includes all promotional efforts before, during, and after the Community Meltdown, such as arranging for print, radio, and television coverage at the local, state, and national levels to encourage participants and other communities to get involved. The media adviser also is responsible for the internal communication networks (Web site, blog, e-mail, etc.). Another dimension of the media adviser's work involves documentation of the Community Meltdown.

The media adviser may disseminate information directly, for example, by sending a press release to a newspaper. (See the appendix for a sample press release.) However, information about the event needs to be disseminated primarily by tapping into existing networks. For example, the media adviser can prepare a promotional flyer or FAQs (frequently asked questions) for e-mail distribution to Weight Watchers members. See the appendix for samples of the promotional flyer and FAQs. The media adviser can also distribute articles on various fitness topics written by Carole Carson along with an alphabetized fitness list. See the appendix for a directory of available articles, a sample article, and "The ABCs of Fitness."

Fitness center liaison: The fitness center liaison solicits cooperation and support from fitness center owners and professionals, disseminates information to them, and solves problems with them as the need arises. Getting support in the form of free passes for Community Meltdown participants is an important part of the liaison's job.

Event producer: The event producer is in charge of all tasks relating to the venue for the sessions and participant comfort at the sessions. He or she works closely with the supervisor of volunteers (described below). Much of the work involves equipment (sound systems, PowerPoint presentation hookups, etc.). A person familiar with the venue and experienced in operating a variety of equipment and systems can save time and keep program presentations running smoothly. The event producer also needs to find ways to include young people in the production of the Community Meltdown, from setting up chairs to handing out bottles of water.

Supervisor of volunteers: The supervisor of volunteers is in charge of recruiting and training volunteers to work at the scheduled sessions—before, during, and after the programs. Depending upon the number of participants, the supervisor may need thirty to fifty volunteers. A service or special-interest group such as a running club or a hiking group is the logical place to find both the supervisor and the needed volunteers. Members typically are already engaged in promoting healthier lifestyles and may welcome the opportunity to play a visible role in helping the entire community address issues of fitness. The supervisor of volunteers also establishes a communication system for volunteer workers. This person works closely with the event producer.

Captain of captains: The captain of captains oversees the network of teams. Depending upon the number of participants, this network may include from one hundred to three hundred teams. During registration and during the sessions, participants are assigned to teams. Each team has a captain. The captain of captains oversees the process of organizing the teams and ensures that each team designates a captain.

The captain of captains also collects statistics and other information from the team captains, consolidates it, and makes the information available to the event organizers. In addition, the captain of captains is the communication link between the teams and the CEO.

Executive assistant to the CEO and/or bookkeeper: One or more people are needed to keep track of the progress of the projects and work assignments of the event organizers and to handle basic bookkeeping. The number of assistants needed depends upon the number of participants in the Community Meltdown. The assistants work closely with the CEO. For ease of administration, we suggest combining the tasks of bookkeeping with those of the executive assistant.

Prize and vendor coordinator: The prize and vendor coordinator works with businesses and donors to obtain prizes for teams. This person plays an integral part in promoting the Community Meltdown and rewarding the success of the participants. Ideally, he or she is resourceful and connected within the community. Prizes and donations may be solicited or volunteered and include products (such as fitness equipment) and services (such as teeth whitening from a dentist). Businesses are likely to continue contributing prizes and donations throughout the event. This is a valuable way for them to express their support for the goal of community fitness, and it involves them in a meaningful way. Each business or organization, however large or small, has the opportunity to make a unique contribution.

Business and legal adviser: The business and legal adviser works closely with the event producer to address any business and legal issues, including risk management. For example, insurance for the venue may be required. Rather than purchase the insurance, the adviser could ask a local insurance broker to donate the needed insurance as a contribution to the Community Meltdown. A word of caution: although a sample legal release and waiver of liability form is provided in the appendix, the business and legal adviser needs to make sure that all forms are in compliance with applicable rules, regulations, and laws.

Medical adviser: The medical adviser is responsible for providing the appropriate medical perspective of the Community Meltdown. The field of fitness is populated with many theories and products that may be unhealthful; consequently, it is important that the medical adviser make sure that information and presentations are grounded in science and provided by responsible, knowledgeable experts. A good candidate for this position would be the wellness coordinator of a local hospital who is familiar with the top talent in the medical community. The medical adviser works closely with the CEO to make sure the content of presentations is accurate, timely, and relevant, as well as to ensure that the presenter has a dynamic style.

Registrar: The duties of the registrar may be performed by the executive assistant to the CEO or separated out, depending upon the size of the event. The registrar works closely with the media adviser and webmaster. The registrar's tasks primarily involve recording and disseminating information about participants for use by the event organizers in planning and delivering programs and publicizing results.

All of the core team members contribute their talents and expertise toward a common goal—helping members of the community and each other lead more healthful lives. Although some people may see obesity as an overwhelmingly intractable problem, these core team members commit themselves to a series of concrete, practical actions that will reverberate beyond their community's boundaries, touching the lives of people in ways they will never know.

Notes

4. Set Goals and Create Structure

People are more fun than anybody.
—DOROTHY PARKER

Once you have articulated the vision, issued an invitation, lined up support, and assigned tasks to the core team, the next step is to set goals and create structure.

Assigning Tasks and Deadlines

The responsibilities of the core group members were summarized in the prior chapter; lists of key tasks (pages 50–63) and actions (pages 82–84) for executing those responsibilities are included in the appendix. A word of caution: the list of action items suggests a sequential process when in fact much of the work must be done concurrently. Progress needs to occur on several fronts, and projects will be accomplished in varying stages. What's important is not whether the linear sequence of tasks is followed (life is a little messier than plans permit) but rather that everyone is making a unique contribution as efficiently and effectively as possible.

To that end, after dividing up work and setting deadlines, the CEO needs to empower the members of the core team to do their jobs with a minimum of intrusion. Close coordination between key players is assumed. In order for the core team to use time efficiently and effectively to achieve that coordination, we recommend communicating via e-mail and telephone whenever possible and eliminating, or at least minimizing, face-to-face meetings.

We also encourage the core team to utilize all of the available resources in the community. Tapping into existing volunteer or fitness groups willing to contribute to the larger effort spreads the workload and has the added benefit of increasing participation. For example, the core team can talk to representatives of medical, religious, and service organizations that may have members who want to promote fitness. These members can be recruited for all sorts of tasks—from directing traffic and parking at sessions to greeting guests at the door.

Establishing Policies

Only a few policies need to be established, announced at the first session, and enforced. The most important policy is that vendors are not allowed to promote weight-loss products or services, with limited exceptions. During sessions, persons who try to promote their businesses in violation of Community Meltdown policies should be asked to leave the venue. Literature and products distributed without authorization need to be destroyed. A flyer covering these basic ground rules must be created and distributed by the event producer before questions arise. Here are some types of allowable promotions:

Presenters: Presenters take their time to give useful information during the sessions. In return for their efforts, they are allowed to offer free classes, distribute brochures, highlight special offers such as a discount on services, and engage in other promotional activities, as approved by the event organizers, at weekly sessions.

Award donors: Donors of prizes for individuals or teams are allowed to distribute material at an approved display site. The display might include literature on discounted services or brochures describing programs offered. Display units need to be staffed by knowledgeable personnel.

Vendors: With the event organizers' approval, vendors may set up tables and give gifts to participants to support nonprofit, charitable efforts. For example, Weight Watchers may give free T-shirts promoting a national weigh-in day in partnership with the National Cancer Society.

Fitness centers: Fitness centers that have donated passes for use by participants during the Community Meltdown are permitted to staff a display at an approved location. Fitness centers can be encouraged to offer special membership promotions at the end of the Community Meltdown.

Health- and wellness-related service providers: Persons providing massages, body-fat testing, blood-pressure testing, and other health- and wellness-related services are allowed to set up tables and distribute literature. Personnel providing services need to be licensed or professionally trained.

A second policy is that eligibility for grand prizes, that is, prizes awarded at the final session, is dependent upon registration and participation for the duration of the Community Meltdown. While grand prizes will probably be known at the start of the program, smaller prizes and donations will likely be given over the course of the event. The smaller prizes can be weekly incentives, and the basis for their award can be assigned each week, depending upon the focus of that week's presentation.

Policies specific to a particular issue (for example, the minimum age for participants) can be established by the core team member responsible for that area (in this example, the registrar).

Setting the Overall Goal

Fitness is an abstract idea; hence, it is difficult to measure. The concept encompasses not only appropriate weight but also elements such as balance, flexibility, strength, vitality, and endurance. The easiest measurement of fitness is weight, although participants who have other goals (increased flexibility, for example) are encouraged to participate.

If your community is typical, being overweight is likely to be a problem for two-thirds of the participants. Weight is a measurement they can relate to and also report easily; hence, our recommendation is that the overall goal be set for pounds lost. Other measurements, such as body mass index and waist circumference, are difficult to measure accurately in a large group or are too variable by body type. Goals beyond or in addition to weight loss can be accommodated at the team level, which is covered in the next chapter.

A reasonable goal is 1 pound per person per week. If a thousand people participate for seven weeks, then a reasonable goal might be a weight loss of 7,000 pounds. In the case of the Nevada County Meltdown, over one thousand of us lost 7,509 pounds in seven weeks.

Setting the Duration

The prevailing wisdom is that changing a habit requires a fair amount of time—between four and eight weeks. Because the overall goal of the Community Meltdown is to help participants learn healthier habits (and give up dysfunctional ones), the suggested length is a minimum of six weeks. The duration is also designed to be long enough for bonding to occur among teammates so that they will continue to provide support long after the Community Meltdown has ended.

We suggest limiting the program to seven weeks, which results in eight sessions. Commitments longer than this are difficult to sustain. The first session is used to organize teams and set a collective goal. The six middle sessions focus on program goals. The eighth and final session is celebratory.

Deciding on the Time of Year

Each time of year has opportunities and drawbacks. January suggests New Year's resolutions—a time to begin anew—but winter weather may make travel difficult in some parts of the country. Spring triggers the impulse for a fresh beginning and reminds us that the summer swimsuit season is just around the corner. But the habit of winter cocooning may be difficult to break.

Summertime creates opportunities for outdoor exercising, such as taking a walk at sunset or going for a swim in a pool; however, excessive heat in some regions may make it difficult or even dangerous to exercise outdoors. Fall triggers memories of returning to school and learning new lessons. The rush of back-to-school life, however, sometimes makes it hard for parents to participate.

The advent of the holiday season (from Halloween to New Year's Day) reminds us that if we don't make changes, we'll end the year with yet a few more pounds added from holiday fare. This busy season, though, makes it especially hard for people to squeeze in other commitments.

Be assured that you will face obstacles whatever time you choose to create your Community Meltdown. You can also be assured that "now" will never seem to be the right time. It is, however, the only time we have.

Scheduling Sessions

We recommend that participants gather weekly to celebrate their achievements, reconnect with each other, and recommit to their goals. Attendance at sessions is not required but strongly encouraged.

Sessions for the Nevada County Meltdown were held on weekday nights so that persons who worked at daytime jobs could participate. Tuesdays were selected because many members of the community had commitments on other nights. For your Community Meltdown, depending upon the preferences of your community, you could also consider scheduling sessions on weekends or during weekdays. Parallel sessions (one in the daytime for those who are unable to attend nighttime sessions as well as an evening session for those who work weekdays) could also be scheduled.

The formal programs for the Nevada County Meltdown were limited to one hour and fifteen minutes and began promptly at 7:00 PM. Pre-event activities began ninety minutes before the formal program. Teams were encouraged to use this time to meet informally, exercise, and to provide encouragement to each other. Each week, we encouraged participants to bring new participants. Consequently, we formed and added teams each week.

For event organizers comfortable with a more formal structure, the lack of strict boundaries for the Community Meltdown may be troubling. Be assured that the program is intentionally designed to be fluid and flexible. Keep in mind that the purpose of the Community Meltdown is not to keep track of people but rather to get people on track, recognizing that the real work of achieving and maintaining fitness begins when the Community Meltdown ends.

Notes

5. Establish Accountability

Just don't give up trying to do what you really want to do.
Where there is love and inspiration, I don't think you can ever go wrong.

—ELLA FITZGERALD

Accountability relies on communication. We monitor our results through feedback and can then make the necessary corrections. Feedback also helps us celebrate our successes and recommit to our goals. Consequently, a successful Community Meltdown requires the creation of an electronic "village"—a series of networks whose members work voluntarily and cooperatively to accomplish a shared goal. To be effective, the village must be organized so that the members and leaders can communicate easily and efficiently. By constantly exchanging information, the participants create an intentional feedback loop, thereby holding one another accountable.

Five categories of networks must be created to ensure that speedy communications can occur both laterally and vertically, internally and externally. The primary focus needs to be on e-mail because it allows village members to communicate and get feedback with minimal delay.

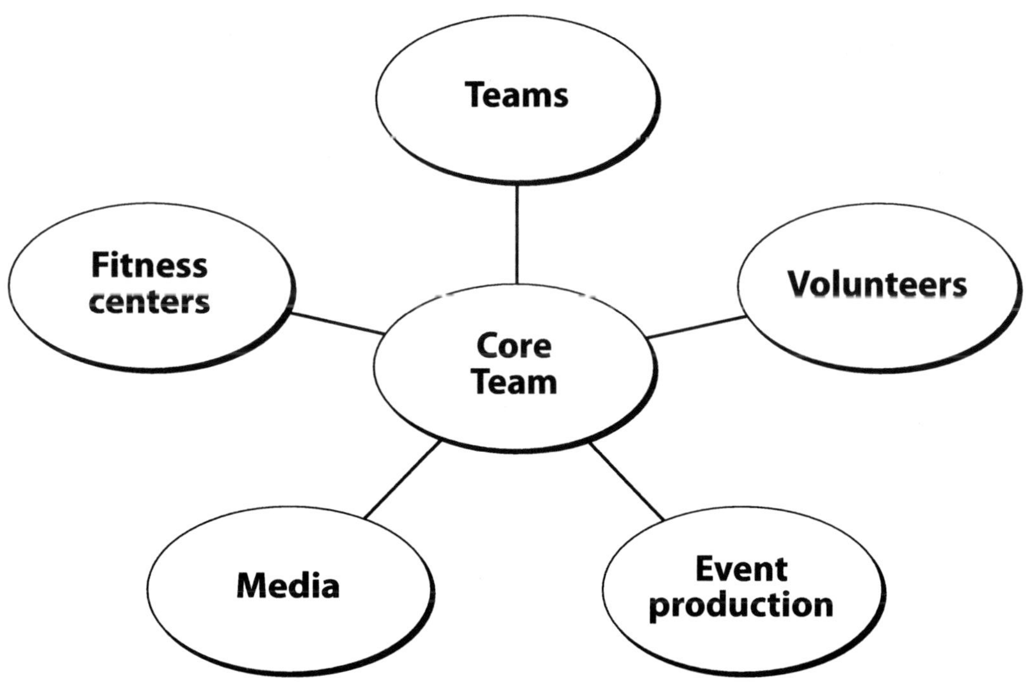

The Five Major Communication Networks

The interactive communication networks can be used for reporting and disseminating individual, team, and group results. Publicly acknowledging victories has a synergistic effect. A dedicated Web site and multiple communications through local television, radio, and newspapers bring the effort into the public arena, creating even more accountability. The event organizers can create a community blog or forum where individuals and teams can share stories, exchange recipes, arrange clothes exchanges, challenge other teams, ask about resources, find a team to join, and arrange rides to sessions. This public dialogue reinforces the participants' obligation to support and encourage each other.

The five major communication networks are described below.

Teams

The key to a successful Community Meltdown is having teammates who cheer each other on and hold each other accountable. Teams are at the heart of the Community Meltdown; hence, the primary communication network consists of teams, each of which has at least one participant.

Teams are formed two ways. Some will form before the first session based on prior affiliations, such as church membership or employment. A few will consist of family members. The majority of teams, however, will form at the first session. A team registration form given to the registrar makes a team's participation official. The registration form may be submitted in advance of the first session, at the first session, or, for new teams, at subsequent sessions. See the appendix for a sample team registration form.

During the formation of teams at the first session, participants are grouped by one or more categories, such as proximity (neighbors), daytime exercisers, walkers and hikers, church membership, fitness center membership, employer, and so on. These larger groups are then broken down into smaller groups (four to six participants) and assigned to a team. Establishing competitions between rival organizations or businesses, such as a team of bank employees competing against a team from a rival bank, adds another dimension to the Community Meltdown.

Once everyone has been assigned to a team, volunteers who have been trained as team facilitators help the newly formed groups get organized.

A facilitator takes each group through a series of questions designed to help members bond into a team. The facilitator also reviews the roles and responsibilities of the captain and teammates. The facilitator encourages the team to pick a unique name and come to sessions in costumes or uniforms.

The facilitator works with the team members until they have picked a captain, set their goals, established an internal system of communication, scheduled their weekly reporting, reviewed their roles and responsibilities, and so on. See the appendix for samples of a team formation checklist and a list of the roles and responsibilities of team captains and teammates.

Although there is no minimum or maximum limit to the size of teams, we recommend teams of five people for ease of communication. Teammates share their phone numbers, e-mail addresses, exercise routines, recipes, progress, relapses, and progress after a relapse. The team captain consolidates the pertinent information and reports it to the captain of captains on a weekly basis.

Assuming that weight loss is the goal chosen for your Community Meltdown, the team captains need to gather information on the starting weight of their team. After the initial weight report, the teammates report their current weight to their captain on a weekly basis. The captains total the weight and report the collective team weight to the captain of captains. This reporting system assures accountability within teams and simultaneously conveys a sense of contributing to a larger purpose. See the appendix for a sample weekly reporting form.

How and where teammates measure their weight is a matter of their own choosing. For consistency's sake, we suggest that participants weigh in at the same time each week wearing similar clothes.

Team captains are required to report their statistics the day before each weekly session. The captain of captains and the event organizers must emphasize the importance of meeting the weekly deadline. Setting and enforcing a consistent deadline makes everyone's job easier. With the weight information e-mailed on time and at the same time each week, the captain of captains can tabulate and present results at the next session, thereby reinforcing accountability.

The captain of captains calculates each team's losses (or gains) by comparing the total current weight with that of the reported weight from the prior week. The captain of captains summarizes the information and makes it available on the Web site, to media, and most importantly, to participants at the following session. See the appendix for a sample summary statistical reporting form.

The captain of captains or CEO can send e-mails to individuals, teams, and the larger community as needed. These communications may include results, ideas, plans, anecdotes, announcements, and so on. Once again, the purpose is to encourage accountability by publicizing results, thereby encouraging further progress.

Media

The media network consists of two parts: external and internal. For external communications, the media adviser needs to compile a list of contacts (print, radio, television, Web sites, etc.) and establish relationships through which information can be disseminated. The media adviser needs to create a network of participants who are willing to be interviewed by media and locations that can serve as backgrounds for coverage, such as restaurants with special menus and fitness centers with special programs.

Because messages in different media reach different audiences, the media adviser needs to stream results, anecdotes, and useful fitness information to a variety of outlets. Receiving multiple messages (for example, hearing an announcement on the radio, seeing a television clip, and reading about the Community Meltdown in a newspaper and a church bulletin) gives legitimacy to the effort and creates momentum. The momentum in turn translates into accountability regarding results.

Internally, the media adviser needs to work with the captain of captains and other event organizers to keep participants informed and enthusiastic. One particularly effective tool to accomplish this goal is a Community Meltdown Web site. Working through the webmaster, the media adviser can use the Web site to keep participants current on results.

In addition, the webmaster needs to feature team statistics, resource information, places to post information, a list of places and times for community walks, endorsements, announcements, a list of prizes, recipes, and other helpful information. See the appendix for a sample community fitness resources list featuring free or low-cost exercise facilities and opportunities.

Other internal communication avenues could involve electronic forums or blogs to which participants could contribute.

Fitness Centers

The fitness center liaison needs to encourage trainers and other fitness center staff to establish an internal e-mail network for potential members who participate in the Community Meltdown. This network can be used to offer special programs, promote membership, provide training tips, share inspiring stories, help members find exercise partners, and so on. Fitness center communications need to be especially welcoming, given that some participants may be working out in a fitness center for the first time and may find the environment intimidating. See the appendix for a sample fitness club internal communication to participants.

The fitness center liaison also needs to collect and organize information specific to each location, including the name of the fitness center owner and other contact persons. In order to do so, the liaison needs to compile a list of physical addresses of fitness centers, phone numbers, e-mail addresses, best times to reach contact persons, and a description of the resources available at the sites. This information can be used by the liaison to match participants with the appropriate fitness center and also to keep fitness center staff informed of pertinent developments.

Volunteers

The supervisor of volunteers needs to establish a communication network by compiling a list of volunteers' names, addresses, phone numbers and e-mail addresses; best times to reach the volunteers; and so on. The communication network can be used to inform volunteers of special plans, setup requirements, and unique arrangements for each session. By sending and receiving information through this network, the supervisor of volunteers enhances the experience of those who are giving their time to serve others.

Event Production

The event producer needs to establish a communication network with contact information for everyone involved in production, especially technical advisers who are familiar with the sound and lighting systems of each venue, setup requirements for PowerPoint presentations, and so on. By sending and receiving information through this network, the event producer assures the quality of each session, thereby contributing to the overall results.

In addition to communications within the networks described above, from time to time, an individual participant or team captain may contact an event organizer with questions, concerns, or suggestions. The core team member contacted needs to respond as quickly as possible.

Today's advanced technology makes efficient communication immediately available in most communities. The Community Meltdown systematically harnesses this technology to serve our ends, creating accountability and reinforcing a sense of belonging.

A team is created when a small group of people begin sharing their goals, dreams, and progress. A community is created when those same teams join with each other to reach a common goal. The result of the collective effort is energizing—hundreds of ongoing interactions within and among team members, event organizers, fitness center staffs, the media, and volunteers. Taken together, these communications generate excitement, enthusiasm, and a sense of being part of a larger effort. And when we both give and receive support, our sense of accountability to others is reinforced. Each communication, valuable in itself, ultimately contributes to the successful outcome of the entire event.

Notes

Notes

6. Learn, Experiment, and Celebrate

The universe will reward you for taking risks on its behalf.

—SHAKTI GAWAIN

The celebration of the Community Meltdown includes a series of weekly sessions. During the first session, the vision of what can be accomplished is shared, teams are organized, and basic information on fitness is provided. The second and subsequent sessions celebrate individual, team, and group success and expand on various aspects of fitness education. The final session celebrates individual and collective success stories before moving on to chart the future. This chapter will provide a brief overview of the content and nature of the sessions.

The spokesperson is a likely candidate to serve as master of ceremonies for the sessions; however, the role may be shared with others who have the ability to create a sense of playfulness. Whoever leads the sessions must be enthusiastic and convey high energy. The most important goal of the Community Meltdown is for participants to connect within their community and have fun getting fit.

Preparation for each session is required, but remember to be flexible. Although we refer to evening sessions in this chapter, you might choose to hold some or all of your sessions during the day if that's more convenient for the participants in your community. Here is the overall approach we recommend:

Solicit ideas from the participants. Be open to spontaneity. Encourage playful creativity. Having fun will enrich the effort. Some of the fun and most memorable moments may come from participants' creativity. For example, a team might volunteer to do a skit. Or a woman may decide to do a "striptease" dance, shedding her larger-sized clothing till she's down to her current size. Participants are creating the Community Meltdown just as much as the planners and presenters are.

Keep an experimental outlook. If something works, keep it. If it doesn't, toss it and go on to the next great idea. After each session, the event organizers need to meet and do a quick critique of the evening's program.

Encourage presession activities. These activities can range from blood-pressure testing and a demonstration of tai chi to nutrition counseling. Exercise classes can be offered. Areas for walking can be set aside. All participants who walk into a session need to be greeted with music, high energy, and a range of activities offering many choices.

Give attention to the logistics. The event organizers can enhance team spirit and efficiency by encouraging participants to carpool. Make sure that parking space is adequate and that all venues are easily accessible and familiar to the community. Enlist volunteers to direct traffic and assist with parking.

To ensure comfort for the participants during each session, make sure that seating is adequate and comfortable and that people have room to move around. Also, make sure seating can accommodate larger-sized participants. The event producer needs to do a walk-through of the venue prior to the session, making sure restrooms are clean and well supplied, trash cans are on hand, and extension cords are taped securely to the floor. Depending upon the facility, consider bringing heavy-duty, extra-length extension cords. Make sure free drinking water is available. In addition, consider selling bottled water.

Stay on top of production requirements. The event producer needs to coordinate technical equipment requirements for the session (PowerPoint presentation equipment, sound system, video projector, screen, etc.). The event producer or someone he or she designates needs to be the point person for technical questions.

Make good use of volunteers. The supervisor of volunteers needs to provide his or her workers with written procedures (for setup, breakdown, etc.) and coordinate their activities with the event producer. Volunteers need to arrive two hours before the starting time and wear something that shows they are volunteers, for example, stick-on labels or buttons that say "Ask Me" or T-shirts printed with "Volunteer."

Give prizes frequently and for different reasons. The event organizers are encouraged to be creative in award distribution; the emphasis doesn't have to be solely on weight loss. For example, prizes might be awarded to the youngest or the oldest team, the team with the most spirit, or the individual with the most impact on teammates. Major prizes need to be announced at the beginning of the program and distributed at the final session.

Opening Night: The Kickoff Session

The purpose of the kickoff session is to unite ordinary people who have an interest in getting fit and to share the vision of what can be accomplished together. During the session, teams are organized and basic information is provided. The event organizers need to keep the length of the program to the scheduled time and make sure the media have been invited.

Here are ideas and elements to incorporate into the kickoff program:

1. *Make everyone feel welcome and affirm the Community Meltdown principles.* Volunteer greeters need to welcome each participant. Opening comments need to affirm the three FIT principles of the Community Meltdown: participants are encouraged to have fun, to make individualized choices on how best to eat and exercise, and to participate on a team. Opening comments need to exclude politics, religion, or the sale of any product or service.

2. *Express the vision.* One or more people must provide inspiration by defining the collective vision. Public commitments from prominent members of the community can reinforce this vision.

3. *Establish the collective goal.* Is the goal to lose four tons of weight in eight weeks? Is it to beat the Nevada County Meltdown record?

4. *Provide basic information to help people get started.* Give general information on the problem of obesity and how it affects our lives, why we need to take responsibility for our health, and so on. Information on how to exercise and eat differently also needs to be included.

5. *Create teams.* Team formation can be accomplished in two ways. Some teams will come to the first session already formed; others will need to be formed during the session. However they are formed, teams need to exchange information among members, set goals, pick a captain, and so on.

6. *Explain the ground rules for weekly and final prizes.* Prizes are likely to be added throughout the course of the program, so the basis for weekly awards needs to be readdressed at each session. Distribute incentives for participants to exercise and eat appropriately (for example, passes to gyms and fitness centers) at the conclusion of the kickoff program and announce prizes for the following week.

7. *Get started.* Have scales available for people to use if they want to have their initial weight recorded. Distribute registration forms and explain how to use them. Provide clipboards and extra pens and pencils to fill out the forms. Explain the reporting system and deadline for reporting. Keep the system of reporting weight as simple and clear as possible.

8. *Conduct a question-and-answer period.* The spokesperson needs to allow five to ten minutes for questions. If possible, the event producer needs to provide participants with portable microphones. Volunteers can "run" the microphones to the participants who've indicated they have questions. If portable microphones aren't available, the speaker needs to repeat the question before responding.

9. *Give closing announcements and reminders.* Reminders might include actions to take during the week, such as join a group for a walk, connect with teammates via e-mail, or participate in an exercise class. The spokesperson needs to also announce the topic and speaker for the following session, announce programs and opportunities occurring during the week, and remind participants to report their results to their team captains.

Materials

The registrar brings registration forms and information to each session in anticipation that new participants will continue to join over the course of the event and additional teams will be added to the roster. The executive assistant can assemble and bring copies of other needed forms and materials to each session. The prize coordinator is responsible for bringing awards and incentives, and the captain of captains is responsible for distributing the registration and other forms, clipboards, and pens. See the appendix for a list of materials to bring to sessions.

Crowd Pleasers

Distribute gifts as incentives at the first session. Examples include passes to fitness centers, T-shirts, buttons, and custom water bottles. Don't forget to play uplifting music that ties into the theme of your program. Think of the music as a Community Meltdown soundtrack.

Summary

In summary, during the first session the participants will

- Support and share the vision of the Community Meltdown
- Establish a collective goal
- Learn basic information to get started
- Become part of a team
- Register for the Community Meltdown and sign necessary forms to participate
- Celebrate the FIT principles
- Make friends and have fun

The Show Must Go On: Middle Sessions

The middle sessions celebrate individual, team, and group success and expand on various aspects of fitness education—exercise, eating, medical issues, and so on. The event organizers need to encourage teams to arrive early in order to take advantage of presession activities. For some teams, this time can be used to update each other on their progress. Other teams may use the time to exercise together. Some teams may take advantage of educational and health-screening activities. Keep the length of the formal program within the scheduled time, and make sure the media have been invited.

Here are ideas and elements to work into the middle sessions:

1. *Welcome and congratulate the teams.* Acknowledge them for following through on their commitment to get fit together. Reinforce the sense of teamwork with unifying comments. Highlight the objectives of the Community Meltdown and vision throughout the program, reminding people that fitness is the goal and weight loss is a by-product. Share and celebrate the results to date (for example, collective results, best

team performance, best individual performance). Award weekly prizes to teams and individuals.

2. *Provide open-mike time for participants.* Encourage them to share their testimonials. The Community Meltdown participants are the heart and soul of the program. Their stories can both energize and inspire other participants.

3. *Share announcements.* Let participants know about supplemental programs and promotions that might interest them, such as cooking classes, community walks, free classes for participants, and restaurants with special menus. Update them on future plans. Distribute gifts and incentives, such as free fitness passes. Sell items (buttons, T-shirts, etc.) to promote a sense of identity, unity, and camaraderie. Inform participants of opportunities to talk with the media, and encourage them to share their experiences.

4. *Introduce the guest speaker and presentation topic.* The medical adviser and CEO are responsible for identifying and scheduling presenters for the sessions. Suggested presenters include nutritionists, fitness instructors, physical therapists, medical doctors, lifestyle counselors, and other health and wellness experts. The presenters need to have a clear understanding of the purpose and policies of the Community Meltdown. High energy, credibility, and knowledge of the topic are vital characteristics that the presenter needs to personify.

    To give each fitness topic the attention it deserves, the event organizers need to limit formal presentations to one per session. Presenters should be asked to arrive two hours before the session begins to test the equipment to be used. They need to limit their talk and the question-and-answer period to twenty minutes. Presenters should be encouraged to give participants homework in order to convert abstract ideas to changes in lifestyle.

    Following are topics (and speakers) that may be of interest to participants:

    - Making permanent lifestyle changes (lifestyle counselor)
    - Learning safe, effective body mechanics for everyday tasks (physical therapist)

- Building a home gym for almost nothing (personal trainer)
- Evaluating popular diets and understanding their medical implications (physician)
- Assessing medical risks of obesity (physician or other medical expert)
- Eating healthfully (registered dietitian)

5. *Plan one surprise activity for the session.* For example, use a visual to symbolize how much weight the entire group has lost. In the Nevada County Meltdown, we showcased a vehicle that weighed the same as the total weight lost. Prepare for the unexpected and have fun.

6. *Give closing announcements and reminders.* Homework assignments might tie in with the presentation, such as keeping a food journal, practicing better body mechanics, or trying a new exercise. Reminders might also include actions to take during the week, such as joining a group for a walk, connecting with teammates via e-mail, or trying a new recipe. The spokesperson needs to also announce the topic and speaker for the following session, announce programs and opportunities occurring during the week, and remind participants to report their results to their team captains.

Materials

As previously mentioned, the registrar needs to bring registration forms and information to each session because new participants will want to form teams. The executive assistant can assemble and bring copies of other needed forms and materials. The prize coordinator is responsible for bringing the awards and incentives, and the captain of captains is responsible for distributing the registration and other forms, clipboards, and pens. See the appendix for a list of materials to bring to each session.

Crowd Pleasers

Presession activities may involve health-related services such as blood-pressure testing, exercise opportunities such as a Jazzercise class or demonstration of tai chi, nutritional counseling, and sales of promotional items. Presession activities need to begin at least one hour before the formal program begins. Don't forget to greet participants with upbeat music that reinforces the theme of the program.

Summary

In summary, during each middle session the participants will

- Create synergy with teammates and other participants through acknowledgment of successes
- Better understand the educational components of health and fitness
- Learn about supplemental fitness-related programs offered in the community
- Sign up to speak with the media in support of fitness
- Make friends and have fun

The Grand Finale

The last session celebrates the completion of the Community Meltdown, charts the future, and highlights individual and collective success stories. Once again, presession activities are encouraged to increase participants' enthusiasm. Keep the length of the formal program within the scheduled time, and make sure the media have been invited.

Here are ideas and elements to work into the last program:

1. *Welcome and congratulate the teams for their achievements.* Distribute achievement awards and prizes, including those for most spirited individual or team, best costumes, best team name, oldest team, youngest team, biggest team, and so on. Hold a raffle for the remaining prizes, for which all participants are eligible.

2. *Acknowledge those who have made the Community Meltdown possible.* Distribute prizes and other expressions of appreciation to the captains and event organizers.

3. *Plan a surprise activity.* Find a way to visually represent the group's total weight loss. For example, park a school bus in the front of or inside the venue with a banner that compares the weight of the bus with the total weight lost by participants. Show a video near the end of the session that documents the Community Meltdown. The documentary needs to include as many participants as possible in as

many settings as possible. This video can reinforce the participants' sense of accomplishment.

4. *Bridge to the future.* Concluding comments must stress an ongoing commitment to achieving fitness. Encourage teams to continue to meet and support each other's pursuit of fitness. On a larger scale, based on the theme "The best is yet to come," future programs might include regular community walks and plans for a Community Meltdown reunion.

Materials

Even at the last session, the event organizers need to bring registration forms and information in anticipation of new participants who will want to form teams for future support. The executive assistant can assemble and bring copies of the materials to this session. The prize coordinator is responsible for bringing the awards and incentives, and the captain of captains is responsible for distributing the registration and other forms, clipboards, and pens. See the appendix for a list of materials to bring to this session.

Crowd Pleasers

Presession activities may involve health-related services such as blood-pressure testing, exercise opportunities such as a Jazzercise class or demonstration of tai chi, nutritional counseling, and sales of promotional items. Presession activities need to begin at least one hour before the formal program begins. Once again, the event organizers need to greet participants with upbeat music that reinforces the theme of the Community Meltdown.

Summary

In summary, during the final session, participants will

- Celebrate their individual and collective success
- Experience the impact and empowerment of community
- Leave with resources and networks to help them continue a healthier lifestyle
- Shine for the media
- Make friends and have fun

At the end of the evening, the event organizers can take satisfaction in knowing that their collective efforts had, and will continue to have, an impact on their community and even beyond. The results achieved during the event can be measured, but the majority of the results will show up in years to come and are impossible to measure.

How do you measure the absence of medical problems? Participants may have fewer heart attacks, fewer cases of diabetes, and fewer strokes. Also difficult to measure is the improved quality of life for persons who can now move more freely, have a sense of being in charge of their own well-being and fitness, and feel more connected with neighbors and friends.

In their enthusiasm for these positive changes, participants will spread their message broadly. How do you measure the impact of these communications on family and friends throughout the United States or even the world? Not a single one of us can change without impacting others.

Notes

Notes

7. Advocate Fitness, Health, and Well-Being

From the end spring new beginnings.
—PLINY THE ELDER

The Community Meltdown is intended to create a heightened awareness of the importance of making healthier choices about what we eat and how much we exercise. The event carefully lays the foundation for the next phase of work: encouraging all of us, whatever our age or station in life, to become advocates for fitness, health, and well-being.

Before moving ahead, however, it is necessary to bring closure to the Community Meltdown. To that end, following the final session, the event organizers need to obtain feedback from the participants and groups that contributed to the effort.

Obtaining Feedback

The evaluation process serves several larger purposes. First, giving feedback helps participants put their experience in perspective and hopefully encourages them to continue on their fitness journey. Second, organizers and volunteers who worked hard to make the experience worthwhile receive rewarding feedback. The evaluation also provides valuable information to the event organizers on the aspects and elements that participants found most meaningful. This information can be incorporated into future programs in this community or others.

Participant Evaluations

Using an automated e-mail system, the captain of captains can distribute a questionnaire to each participant. The captain of captains can distribute the tabulated results to event organizers and others as appropriate. Several free survey systems are available on-line. See the appendix for a sample postevent evaluation form.

Fitness Center Evaluations

Fitness centers may wish to measure how many participants became full-time gym members. Collecting data on the conversion rate as well as the data on participation in special programs and classes, use of personal trainers, and so on is helpful in determining the financial viability of participation in future events.

Event Organizers' Critique

A postevent evaluation meeting of the event organizers is also useful. The CEO or the spokesperson needs to invite the core team members to a meeting to assess what was done correctly and what areas could benefit from improvements. This information can be used to help plan future similar programs or be shared with other communities planning similar campaigns.

Don't Quit—Recommit!

Institutionalizing changes is the next big challenge. One person needs to have a continuing role in speaking for fitness in the community and articulating the need for making further changes. This person can serve as a catalyst for pulling people together for future events.

The catalyst can write health- and fitness-related articles for local media, including success stories, and encourage participation at fitness events. In addition, the media adviser needs to find and designate an individual to update the Web site.

The event organizers also need to encourage participants to "sell" fitness, to become actively engaged in the promotion of living a healthy lifestyle. One way to do this is to arrange to have buttons and T-shirts for participants to wear during and after the Community Meltdown. Through continuing efforts, the event organizers need to empower participants to become self-appointed fitness advocates in their own circle of friends, among their neighbors, and in the larger community. The event organizers must encourage participants to contact their elected officials, write to their local newspaper, and make their voices heard in public forums as part of a continuing effort to bring about positive changes.

The event organizers have the task of converting idealism into practical actions. This can take the form of establishing community task forces to bring about positive change in schools, such as healthier food choices for students and increased opportunities for physical exercise. The task force or a similar group could tackle issues involving food served in restaurants, such as posting the caloric content of foods and creating menus that offer healthier choices. The event organizers can also continue to promote fitness through newspaper articles and public service announcements on radio and television, and they can encourage businesses to sponsor and support fitness efforts in the community.

To encourage exercise, the event organizers can initiate community walks and post a calendar of exercise opportunities on the Web site. They can support and encourage fitness programs for children and young adults. The event organizers can also encourage local fitness centers to hold open houses for prospective members and schedule team sports, walks, and fitness programs.

To accomplish this long and varied task list, the event organizers will need to find and associate with persons interested in promoting fitness in the community. Before long, the event organizers will have created a powerful network of people working to create a playful, healthy, and fit community.

Acknowledgments

The CEO needs to send letters of appreciation, including personal notes, to all who played key roles in the success of the Community Meltdown. The prize coordinator needs to send thank-you notes to prize donors. The captain of captains needs to send letters of appreciation to the team captains, and the supervisor of volunteers is encouraged to acknowledge the volunteers.

Networking and Ongoing Leadership

The event organizers need to continue to expand their network of individuals committed to promoting fitness. With this network in place, you will be ready to create an even bigger and better Community Meltdown. The transformation of your community will be complete when being fit is the norm and having fun together is what makes it happen.

To make this vision a reality, we only need to continue. Working together, we can create a future where the best is yet to come!

Notes

Appendix

The appendix serves as your resource center to create and implement a successful Community Meltdown. For the limited purpose of creating your own Community Meltdown, the forms and other materials in this appendix may be copied and distributed. Or you may decide to design material unique to your Community Meltdown.

Information is included that is necessary to organize the Community Meltdown, such as a list of action items, roles and responsibilities, a statistical reporting form, and a weekly reporting form. The promotional materials are suggested tools to publicize your event. Also included is a sample evaluation form.

Producing a Community Meltdown is a group effort involving multiple resources and people. The contents of the appendix are meant to support your endeavors, simplify the process, and encourage fun and creativity.

Sample Proclamation

This sample proclamation can be modified for use by governments at all levels (city, county, state) and can also be used by organizations, agencies, service groups, and employers. The media adviser can arrange for a formal ceremony during the signing of the proclamation in order to trigger newspaper, radio, and television coverage, thereby increasing awareness of the forthcoming sessions.

Resolution In Recognizing January and February 2004 as "Nevada County Meltdown" Months

WHEREAS, four out of five Americans over the age of twenty-five are overweight; and

WHEREAS, four out of five Americans are not meeting the minimum activity level of thirty minutes of exercise per day; and

WHEREAS, one out of four Americans are completely sedentary; and

WHEREAS, since 1990 the medical community has experienced a seventy-six percent increase in diabetes in adults thirty to forty years old; and

WHEREAS, four out of five cases of diabetes are related to obesity; and

WHEREAS, seventy percent of cardiovascular disease is related to obesity; and

WHEREAS, breast and colon cancer, high blood pressure and gall bladder disease are all linked to obesity; and

WHEREAS, the Community Wellness Coalition was formed to identify, develop and support organized community health actions for individual wellness that lead to a healthy community; and

WHEREAS, the Community Wellness Coalition has organized a free community-based event to educate citizens on the value of becoming and remaining fit; and

WHEREAS, professionals in the health and fitness community have volunteered to teach and provide facilities for this event; and

WHEREAS, Nevada County has both the climate and tremendous physical beauty in which to engage in outdoor exercises;

NOW THEREFORE, BE IT RESOLVED, the Board of Supervisors of Nevada County, California, joins with the Community Wellness Coalition in supporting the Nevada County Meltdown throughout Nevada County and encourages the community to participate in this event.

Job Descriptions

Following are the job descriptions of the event organizers. These descriptions can be used as the basis for recruitment and selection of the core team members. They can also be used by the event organizers to guide their daily work.

Spokesperson

Knowledge, skills, and abilities: Knowledge of community resources, decision makers, and leaders. Skill in persuading others to promote fitness, make donations, and support the Community Meltdown in a variety of ways. Ability to attract and manage executive talent. Ability to express a vision of community fitness in terms that inspire individuals and groups, in private and in the public forum. Ability to accomplish tasks with volunteers. Ability to enjoy and create fun whatever the task at hand.

Key tasks:

- Deciding and following through on the decision to create a Community Meltdown
- Picking a name for the event
- Recruiting executives and team members for key roles
- Providing management and supervision
- Organizing work, assigning tasks, and setting deadlines
- Acquiring funding
- Expressing the vision for the Community Meltdown in terms that attract support and participation
- Promoting the Community Meltdown to appropriate media
- Acquiring support from diverse elements in the community, for example, political leaders, fitness center owners, business leaders, healthcare providers, and major employers

Chief Executive Officer

Knowledge, skills, and abilities: Extensive knowledge of the community—its leaders and resources. Skill in working with diverse individuals and groups. Skill in making work assignments fun and enjoyable. Ability to translate an abstract idea, such as a community fitness event, into concrete, practical actions. Ability to build a highly efficient and effective team by working with volunteers.

Key tasks:

- Helping the spokesperson recruit and assemble core team members
- Managing the day-to-day work of producing the Community Meltdown
- Organizing tasks, assigning deadlines, and coordinating the efforts of the event organizers
- Making key policy decisions
- Problem solving and troubleshooting as the need arises
- Coordinating the collection and dissemination of management information
- Leading efforts to promote fitness after the Meltdown officially ends

Media Adviser

Knowledge, skills, and abilities: Knowledge of diverse media contacts and appropriate tools to use for each outlet. Skill in articulating the message in a variety of media (print, radio, television, Web site, blog, and so on). Ability to persuade media contacts and local contacts to promote the Community Meltdown through their unique networks and associations.

Key tasks:

- Promoting the Community Meltdown through local communication networks and making requests for widespread dissemination of the invitation to participate
- Issuing a public challenge (print, radio, television, e-mail networks of various potential endorsers)
- Creating promotional material such as posters, brochures, flyers, and FAQs for use by sponsors or others promoting the Community Meltdown
- Placing articles and other material written by Carole Carson in local print media in order to promote participation
- Developing a press kit and issuing press releases
- Obtaining proclamations from local government bodies and other agencies
- Overseeing the construction of a dedicated Web site, including compiling a list of useful community resources promoting fitness
- Establishing a webmaster to maintain and update the site so that information is always current
- Coordinating appearances of the spokesperson and participants with various media
- Responding to inquiries for information from the media and other communities
- Reviewing printed material distributed on behalf of the event organizers, sponsors, and endorsers
- Preparing individual participants for interviews with the media

- Arranging public service announcements and various forms of endorsements from the media
- Disseminating current statistical progress to the media during the Community Meltdown
- Distilling and disseminating evaluation results at the conclusion of the Community Meltdown
- Arranging for each session to be videotaped or otherwise documented both for historical purposes and for use during the final presentation

Fitness Center Liaison

Knowledge, skills, and abilities: Knowledge of local fitness center owners and their facilities, personnel, and programs. Skill in persuading fitness center owners to support and participate in the Community Meltdown, including donating passes to participants. Skill in helping fitness centers respond to the influx of participants who may be new to exercising. Ability to problem solve with fitness center owners as the need arises.

Key tasks:

- Organizing information about the fitness centers, for example, the names of owners and trainers, locations, hours, programs, available equipment and resources, and policies
- Obtaining free fitness passes and other fitness incentives for participants
- Assisting fitness center owners to schedule and provide appropriate educational programs for Community Meltdown participants
- Visiting fitness centers to encourage owners' participation in the event
- Advising fitness center owners on appropriate internal communication with participants
- Coordinating media coverage with local fitness centers
- Seeking endorsements from fitness center owners for purposes of promoting the Community Meltdown
- Problem solving when special issues arise between participants and fitness center owners
- Coordinating the evaluation of the Community Meltdown by fitness center owners and providing feedback when the evaluation is completed

Event Producer

Knowledge, skills, and abilities: Knowledge of venues in the community, their availability, and their features. Skill in figuring out technical requirements of presentations, seating arrangements, parking requirements, and other aspects of large group sessions. Ability to problem solve and coordinate the work of volunteers.

Key tasks:

- Partnering with the CEO to schedule sessions
- Establishing a production network crew of committed volunteers and maintaining a list with contact information, availability, technical skills, and so on
- Locating and reserving a venue adequate for the needs of the event organizers, including seating, restrooms, parking, lighting, sound system, and so on
- Obtaining keys to the venue and maintaining security for the venue
- Ensuring that necessary business and liability insurance has been obtained for the venue
- Responding to technical requirements of presenters (slide projector, sound system, etc.)
- Determining the procedures for opening and closing the venue for each session and conveying the procedures to the supervisor of volunteers for implementation
- Working with vendors who may be setting up exhibits or providing services before, during, or after weekly sessions; answering questions; and reviewing policies
- Collaborating with the CEO to plan sessions that may have specialized technical requirements
- Overseeing the setup and breakdown for sessions through close cooperation with the supervisor of volunteers
- Overseeing parking and supplying directional signs to the supervisor of volunteers and his or her crew
- Arranging accommodations for the specialized needs of participants, for example, obtaining a sign language interpreter for the hearing impaired

Supervisor of Volunteers

Knowledge, skills, and abilities: Knowledge of service organizations and key leaders in the community. Skill in recruiting and training volunteers. Ability to inspire others to give freely in support of the Community Meltdown. Ability to organize work, set deadlines, and effectively supervise people with a range of personalities.

Key tasks:

- Recruiting volunteers to work on all aspects of the Community Meltdown, including scheduled sessions
- Collecting and maintaining information about volunteers, such as names, addresses, e-mail addresses, phone numbers, expertise, and assignments
- Organizing and delegating volunteers' duties at sessions, such as greeting people, organizing teams, answering participants' questions, setting up and removing furniture, distributing printed material, directing traffic, operating lights, cleaning up, and securing the site
- Writing procedures for specialized volunteer tasks, such as team facilitators' roles and responsibilities during the formation of teams, and training these volunteers for their tasks. (Note: Facilitators are assigned the task of helping individuals, some of whom will be strangers, bond into teams. At the initial session, facilitators will organize most of the teams; however, facilitators need to be present at subsequent sessions as additional teams continue to be formed.)
- Collecting and disseminating feedback from event organizers and volunteers on how to make sessions run more smoothly

Captain of Captains

Knowledge, skills, and abilities: Knowledge of small-group dynamics and ability to inspire others to action. Knowledge of Excel and how to collect, organize, and display statistical information. Skill in managing and synthesizing large amounts of data coming from a variety of sources. Ability to set deadlines and persuade participants to meet those deadlines. Ability to write reports, articles, and other material useful to participants and the general public. Ability to work under the pressure of deadlines for reporting.

Key tasks:

- Ensuring each team has a captain
- Distributing registration and release forms to team captains
- Reporting the teams' progress, concerns, and anecdotes to the event organizers and others who need to be updated
- Making announcements at sessions
- Informing team captains about future plans, changes, and opportunities through an e-mail network and encouraging team captains to share this information with their teammates
- Writing articles and features promoting participation for inclusion in newspapers and the Community Meltdown Web site
- Making appearances as a featured guest for the media
- Encouraging teams to seek endorsements within their own networks
- Partnering with the CEO and registrar to collect testimonial letters from participants

Executive Assistant to the CEO and/or Bookkeeper

Knowledge, skills, and abilities: Knowledge of standard office procedures, bookkeeping principles, and computer systems. Skill in organizing work—one's own and others'. Ability to respond effectively under pressure to people with diverse personalities and competing priorities. Ability to set a lighthearted, playful tone in the office.

Key tasks:

- Partnering with the CEO to complete administrative tasks and scheduling
- Arranging tie-ins with other activities, such as parades, fitness programs, and community walks
- Tracking income and expenses of the Community Meltdown
- Providing information as requested and synthesizing information for others' use
- Tracking projects, deadlines, and assigned tasks and reporting problems, opportunities, or unexpected issues that need to be addressed
- Problem solving with event organizers
- Bringing needed materials to sessions and arranging for copying and distribution
- Overseeing phone communications, responding to e-mails, and speaking for the spokesperson or CEO in his or her absence

Prize and Vendor Coordinator

Knowledge, skills, and abilities: Knowledge of community resources, donors, and key leaders in service and business organizations. Skill in acquiring prizes and incentives for participants. Ability to persuade individuals and organizations to promote fitness through donation of valuable goods and services. Ability to keep records.

Key tasks:

- Obtaining and cataloguing prizes for teams and individuals
- Working with the CEO to determine the criteria and rules for participants' awards
- Soliciting donations of products and service discounts, such as printing, paper, T-shirts and buttons, cookbooks, free passes, and balloons
- Seeking endorsements from the business community and soliciting funding to cover the expenses of the Community Meltdown
- Working with the CEO to order promotional items for the Community Meltdown

Business and Legal Adviser

Knowledge, skills, and abilities: Knowledge of applicable rules, regulations, and laws for the Community Meltdown. Skill in recognizing risks and liabilities and taking proactive steps to avoid problems. Ability to create practical solutions to complex legal and business issues. Ability to explain policies to vendors and others participating in the Community Meltdown in such a way as to promote participation.

Key Tasks:

- Drafting policies and reviewing written contracts that may be entered into on behalf of the event organizers
- Securing necessary insurance for the Community Meltdown
- Preparing a release and waiver of liability for participants in compliance with applicable laws, rules, and regulations
- Articulating and disseminating the ground rules on promotion policies to vendors, presenters, and participants

Medical Adviser

Knowledge, skills, and abilities: Knowledge of medical issues associated with obesity and lifestyle choices. Knowledge of articulate experts in the community in various disciplines, such as physicians, physical therapists, lifestyle counselors, and dietitians. Skill in working with individuals whose specialties span the range of conventional and alternative disciplines.

Key tasks:

- Working with the CEO to identify topics for the educational presentations at sessions
- Interviewing, selecting, and scheduling appropriate speakers
- Reviewing speakers' presentations, ensuring that sales pitches for services are excluded
- Monitoring the content of each session and inserting corrections during the program where needed
- Persuading speakers to offer special programs and services to participants as follow-ups to the presentations
- Writing articles on lifestyle changes, the importance of healthful eating, and exercising regularly for dissemination to various media
- Appearing as the medical expert as needed by the media adviser for interviews in various media

Registrar

Knowledge, skills, and abilities: Knowledge of computer and software systems, collection and organization of data, and forms design. Skill in collecting, distilling, and disseminating information from a variety of sources. Ability to keep reporting systems simple and understandable. Ability to set and maintain deadlines.

Key tasks:

- Establishing a Web-based system for registration and participation
- Tracking information and statistics (names of teams, names of captains, e-mail addresses of participants, number of participants, starting weight, pounds lost, etc.) for registered teams
- Overseeing the distribution and collection of registration forms, waivers, and release of liability forms for all participants
- In support of the media adviser, maintaining a contact list of participants who are willing to talk to the media
- Establishing a cutoff time for weekly reporting of information, including weight-loss information
- Distributing answers to frequently asked questions
- Compiling information for use by the event organizers, such as weight-loss updates, demographics, number of teams, and sizes of teams
- Partnering with the webmaster and the CEO to create and distribute a questionnaire for evaluation of the Community Meltdown
- Disseminating results of the survey to various audiences, such as the CEO, other core team members, team captains, fitness center owners, and the media
- Partnering with the CEO and captain of captains to collect testimonial letters from participants during and after the Community Meltdown for use by the media adviser

Sample Press Release

Following are tips on writing and distributing a press release. Although an experienced media adviser might not need these guidelines, we've included the checklist and sample as a safety net.

- ☐ Cover the five Ws: who, what, when, where, and why.
- ☐ Be brief, accurate, and clear.
- ☐ Include the date and contact information (name, phone number, and e-mail address).
- ☐ Keep radio station press releases very short, generally four or five typed lines.
- ☐ Plan on one to two pages double spaced for newspaper press releases.
- ☐ Timing is everything, so allow yourself sufficient lead time for getting the press release into outlets. Give the release to magazines and newsletters three to four weeks ahead of time; a week or ten days is sufficient for newspapers and radio stations.
- ☐ Contact your local chamber of commerce for a list of organizations, many of which send newsletters to their members. Ask these organizations to include the press release in their next newsletter.
- ☐ Distribute press releases by mail, fax, or e-mail.

See the sample press release on the next page.

FOR IMMEDIATE RELEASE

January 15, 2004

Contact: Carole Carson
PO Box 2328
Nevada City, CA 95959
(530) 478-5709
Carole@HoundPress.com

Community Meltdown: Want to lose 8,000 pounds with your friends and family in less than 8 weeks? Get fit for free and have fun.

Three quarters of us in America are overweight, and the rate of childhood obesity is increasing at an alarming rate. As a community we are taking charge of our well-being and getting fit together. We are organizing a Community Meltdown challenge and you are invited.

The first session is taking place on January 30, 2004, at the Best High School, 123 West Street, Hometown, CA, 6:00 PM–7:30 PM.

Carpooling is encouraged. The Community Meltdown is free. Contact Carole Carson for more information or to volunteer at (530) 478-5709 or Carole@HoundPress.com.

Sample Promotional Flyer

A general information flyer can be created and distributed by the event organizers. Simultaneously, the various businesses, organizations and community groups that may be participating (for example, fitness centers, Weight Watchers, businesses, medical associations) can distribute their own version of the flyer. No matter what the source of the flyer is, each flyer needs to include what the Community Meltdown is, why it is happening, where it is taking place, when it is occurring, and who is sponsoring it. Distribute it to local media outlets, fitness clubs, community networks, local merchants, and friends.

You can take charge of your well-being! There's no time better than NOW!

Imagine if you ate foods that were good for you.
Imagine if you took the time to get enough exercise.
Imagine if you really took care of yourself and your family.
Imagine the benefits, both as an individual
and as a community.

A NEVADA COUNTY HEALTH & WELLNESS EVENT
Meltdown Challenge

MELTDOWN CHALLENGE

Start your New Year off RIGHT! Learn how to exercise effectively and lose weight safely!

The Meltdown is a Community Event designed to help people accomplish their health, exercise and weight loss goals for 2004.

Learn from Nevada County experts in health and fitness for one night each week for 8 weeks. Theory will be combined with practice—non-member participants have free access to exercise facilities at South Yuba Club, Club Sierra, Courthouse Athletic Club, Curves, Fast and Fit during the program.

WHEN

Tuesday, January 6th from 7pm to 9pm. Continues every Tuesday from 7pm to 9pm through February 26th.

WHERE

Bring your questions and commitment to:

South Yuba Club
555 Searls Ave.
Nevada City, CA 95959 **470-9100**

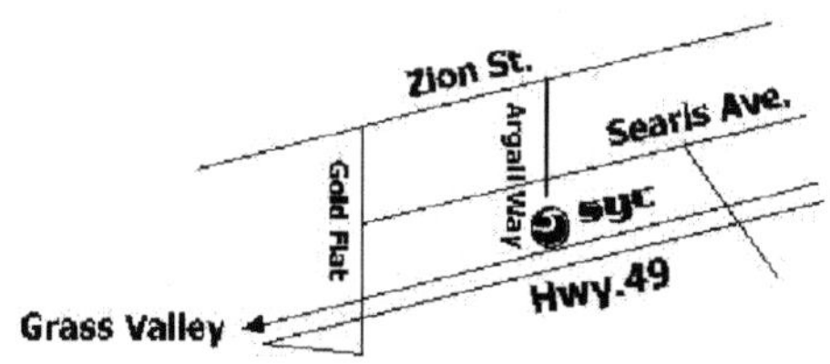

This is a FREE community event!

Brought to you by
CONCERNED LEADERS AND EXPERTS IN THE NEVADA COUNTY FITNESS AND HEALTH COMMUNITY INCLUDING

Community Wellness Coalition

south yuba club

United Way

THE UNION

Sierra Nevada Memorial Hospital

NEVADA COUNTY SUPERINTENDENT OF SCHOOLS

For more information go to

www.southyubaclub.com(as of 12/17)

Sample FAQs

The Community Meltdown may trigger almost as many questions as there are participants. For efficiency in responding to inquiries, a list of frequently asked questions needs to be compiled and answered. The media adviser distributes FAQs to interested parties when the Community Meltdown is announced, thereby saving the registrar considerable time in responding to individual inquiries.

Where the questions are more general, we've included suggested responses. For specific responses, such as locations, dates, and times, you will need to create your own answers.

1. **When does it start? End?**
2. **Who is organizing it?**
3. **Where is the first session being held?**
4. **Who is paying for it?**
5. **What is the goal of the teams?**
   To become fit, have fun, and, as a by-product, lose weight if needed.
6. **Do participants have to attend every session? What if a participant has to miss a session?**
   Attendance at the first session is required to become an official participant. Official participants are eligible for prizes and will be given, upon request, passes to participating gyms/fitness centers. If individuals do not care about prizes or obtaining passes to gyms/fitness centers, they can attend sessions based on convenience and personal preference.
7. **If a participant can't attend the first session, can the participant still be part of the Community Meltdown?**
   Guests are welcome at all of the sessions, but only registered participants are eligible for prizes.
8. **Do all of my teammates have to attend the opening session, or can one or more teammates represent the group?**
   All persons who want to be eligible for prizes and/or obtain passes need to be at the first session. After that, attendance is encouraged but not required.
9. **What are the prizes?**
   The most important prize is a more fit you. Prizes donated by individuals and organizations will be announced at the first session. Additional prizes will be announced over subsequent sessions as they are received by the event organizers.
10. **Do all of my teammates have to exercise in the same way? at the same time? at the same location?**
    No. Team members can work out individually or however they want, whenever they want.
11. **Do I need to work out at a gym to participate?**
    Absolutely not. Exercise comes in many forms—dancing, fencing, walking, gardening, skateboarding, and more. We will encourage participants to exercise in ways that are safe and fun and appropriate for each.

12. **What should I wear to sessions? Will we be exercising?**
Dress comfortably. We will not be exercising unless you count clapping, laughing, or yelling!

13. **Are there any age restrictions?**
Official participants need to be eighteen or older. There is no upper limit.

14. **Can my children come with me to weekly sessions?**
Yes, as long as they are twelve years or older and won't disturb others. Only persons eighteen or older, however, will be officially registered.

15. **Can my family members be on my team?**
Yes, but again, only family members eighteen or older will be officially registered.

16. **What if I don't know anyone who wants to be a part of a team?**
We'll be matching people with others who need to join a team on the first night.

17. **Can I be a team of one? Or can we have more than five people on a team?**
You can be a team of one or have a team of twenty. For purposes of awarding prizes, however, we'll have to limit the competition to five people. A team of ten, for example, may want to have their best five people compete for prizes.

18. **Do teammates have to be overweight and out of shape to join?**
No. Everyone who wishes to focus on fitness is welcome. We expect to have some participants join to support their spouses or other teammates. Others will be addressing issues of flexibility or strength.

19. **What happens when the Community Meltdown is over?**
We'll work together to find ways to continue our focus on fitness.

20. **Do I have to tell people what I weigh?**
Your team captain will need to know at the beginning and then again each week. Otherwise, we can't measure the losses and give prizes. But remember, Carole Carson had her full 182 pounds listed on the front page of her local newspaper. What could be worse than that?

)(

An ounce of action
is worth a ton of theory.

FRIEDRICH ENGELS

)(

Directory of Articles

Carole Carson has written nearly three hundred published articles in which she has shared her insights and personal experience as she traveled on her fitness journey. These articles are available to your community to promote fitness. Contact Carole at Carole@HoundPress.com for a complete list of the available articles. In addition, if you want an article on a specific health or fitness topic, let her know.

Included in this appendix is a sample article written by Carole, "Hot Tubbing with a Frog: The Danger of Postponing Getting Fit." To pique interest, you may want to distribute this and other articles to potential participants a month or two prior to initiating your Community Meltdown. You may want to continue to use the articles during the sessions to reinforce the notion of promoting fitness. Carole's articles also may be submitted to local media outlets (for example, radio stations, newspapers, television stations) and e-mailed to parties of interest.

Here is a list of articles ready and available for your use:

- **Hot Tubbing with a Frog: The Danger of Postponing Getting Fit**
- **Timing: Are You Ready?**
- **UFOs: Unexpected Fitness Obstacles**
- **Crises: Our Own and Others'**
- **Eating: What about Food?**
- **Children: The Expanding Problem of Obesity**
- **Exercise: Learn to Play and Have Fun**
- **Alternatives: Beyond the Treadmill**
- **Pitfalls: Bad Advice**
- **Intelligent Design: Use Your Head**
- **Fitness Benefits: Why Bother?**
- **Insights: Tips and Creative Ideas**
- **Medical Issues: Injuries and Conditions**
- **Recruiting: Spreading the Word**
- **Sustaining Commitment: Avoiding or Recovering from Relapses**
- **Resources: Information and Research**
- **Profiles: Recent Converts or "Lifetimers"**

Sample Article

Event organizers are encouraged to distribute this article to potential participants through publication in newspapers, newsletters, employee communications, Web sites, blogs, and other forms of written communication. The intent is to lift up for public discussion a matter that is privately troubling to many people. By exposing her own struggles, Carole opens up the possibility of change. If, as an ordinary person, she could lose weight and get fit, others could follow in her steps.

Hot Tubbing with a Frog: The Danger of Postponing Getting Fit

Carole Carson

Do you remember the science experiment with the frog and hot water? How if you put a frog in boiling water, he'll hop out? But if you put the frog in cold water and heat the water gradually, he'll remain until, alas, it is too late! The boiling water will kill him.

The experiment illustrates two points: First, conditions that would be intolerable if confronted in their entirety can be accommodated when introduced incrementally. I would not, for example, voluntarily carry around a sixty pound sack of bricks. Yet I had no problem acquiring a pound or two a year until I reached 182 pounds.

Second, in accommodating small changes, we passively participate in our own demise. At the time I decided to get fit, I was prompted by embarrassment and shame at my appearance. In retrospect, however, I wonder if a primitive instinct for survival was whispering in my ear that if I didn't shape up, I wouldn't have a future.

Whatever my reasons, before being lulled into total unconsciousness and while I still could, I jumped out of the slowly heating water and began my fitness program.

Make Changes While You Still Can

Debbie Wagner, R. N. and Lifestyle Counselor, encourages individuals "to make changes while you still can. By the time you decide to change, the window of opportunity may be closed or at least closing. For example, back or joint problems from years of carrying around extra weight make exercise painful. Increased pain leads to a more sedentary lifestyle that leads to more weight gain."

She adds, "Although the effects aren't noticed on a single day, lack of exercise and increased weight contributes to heart disease, stroke, and cancer. Rather, the damage silently accumulates over time until past decisions create irreversible medical problems."

In my "BC" period ("Before Conditioning"), I loved anything round and greasy! Losing weight meant I'd have to go without. Exercise was a burden on top of an already heavy workload.

Silly me! I had it backwards. Deprivation isn't giving up that chocolate sundae before retiring. It's giving up a walk because of joint pain or lack of energy. Deprivation isn't going without sausage pizza and beer. It's going without self-esteem when you look in the mirror.

Deprivation isn't about scheduling time in the coming week for exercise. It's when you don't have a future to look forward to.

Having made the decision to jump out of hot water, it would, you'd think, be permanent. Yet the pivotal decision is only the start. Each day, I must decide what to eat and whether or not to exercise.

One Day at a Time

Getting sidetracked is easy, particularly during special occasions or traveling when we are encouraged to indulge. When it comes to fitness, though, there are only two conditions: in hot water or outside hopping around.

Either I'm keeping my covenant to live healthily, or I'm contributing to my demise. Either I'm being a responsible steward in caring for my body, or I'm abusing it with insufficient rest, too much food or not enough exercise. Either I'm making progress, or I'm losing ground.

Knowing the number of decisions that lie ahead could be daunting, if I let it be. Instead, I find the ongoing process reassuring. Past decisions don't control the future. If I mistakenly get into hot water, I can quickly hop back out!

William James said: "The greatest discovery of my generation is that a human being can alter his life by altering his attitudes of mind."

Seeing deprivation for what it really is has altered my attitude. Deprivation isn't giving up a second helping. Real deprivation is losing the freedom to live life to its fullest because of being overweight and lack of fitness. Deprivation is transformed into personal freedom.

If you've made the leap of faith, congratulations! If you're thinking about it, hurry, it's not too late! The water's getting hotter!

The ABCs of Fitness

This list can be printed on the backs of flyers and published in newspapers, newsletters, Web sites, blogs, and other written communications.

The ABCs of Fitness

Appreciate your body

Begin today

Commit for a lifetime

Delay gratification

Expect obstacles

Forgive lapses

Give up excuses

Have a plan

Individualize your program

Journal daily

Keep learning

Listen to yourself

Make it fun

Notice improvement

Open your heart

Play and laugh

Quit procrastinating

Review and revise

Seek help

Tell others

Underscore success

Vaporize saboteurs

Watch portion size

Xercise daily

Yell "no" to dieting

Zero in on a healthy lifestyle

Sample Legal Release for Participants

Although the possibility of a lawsuit is remote, it is still prudent to get a release and waiver of liability signed by each participant. This release and waiver also gives event organizers permission to publicize information about the Community Meltdown involving participants. Please make sure that your legal adviser reviews this sample and makes the necessary corrections to assure compliance with applicable laws, rules, and regulations.

RELEASE AND WAIVER OF LIABILITY FOR PARTICIPANTS

Please read this document carefully.
By signing it, you are giving up legal rights.

In consideration for being permitted to participate in the ________________ Community Meltdown™ and activities related thereto (collectively, "Activities"), both today and in the future, the undersigned hereby agrees as follows:

ASSUMPTION OF RISK: I am, and/or my child/ward is, voluntarily participating in the Activities. I assume, on behalf of myself and/or my child/ward, all risk of personal injury, death or disability to me and/or my child/ward that might result from said Activities, or any damage, loss or theft of any personal property which I or my child/ward may incur. I understand that the Activities include weight loss suggestions and ideas, suggestions for exercise and other physical activities, and that these have inherent risks. I have been advised that it is strongly recommended that participants in the Activities consult with their doctor or other qualified medical practitioner before engaging in the Activities.

I understand and accept the above risks of bodily injury and property loss related to the Activities. ________ (INITIALS)

RELEASE OF LIABILITY: On behalf of myself and/or my child/ward and my/their personal representatives, successors, heirs, and assigns, I expressly release and discharge the organizers of the Activities, Baskerville Enterprises, Hound Press and their affiliates, leaders, officers, managers, agents, employees, volunteers and members, as well as any person or entity who provides low cost or free services to participants in the Activities, and their managers, agents, employees and owners (collectively, the "Released Parties") from any and all liability, claims, demands or causes of action whatsoever arising out of any personal injury, disability, or death, and any damage or loss to me and/or my child/ward or our property, while participating in any of the Activities. This release is valid and effective whether the damage, loss, injury or death is a result of any act or omission on the part of a Released Party or from any other cause, even if negligence is involved on the part of a Released Party. This Waiver and Release of all liability includes, without limitation, injuries, illness, accidents or loss which may occur as a result of (a) engaging in any Activity; (b) exercise or other strenuous bodily movement; (c) instruction or supervision; or (d) slipping and falling while attending a session of the Community Meltdown or on the premises during a session of a Community Meltdown event.

On behalf of myself and/or my child/ward and my/their personal representatives, successors, heirs, and assigns, I further expressly agree not to sue the Released Parties for any claim, injury, liability, cause of action, expense, damages or other matter that may arise from my participation in the Activities. I agree that if I do file suit, I will be responsible for all costs and expenses incurred by the Released Parties in defending the suit, including without limitation court costs and reasonable attorneys' fees.

I understand that I voluntarily give up any claims I may have, now or in the future, against the Released Parties, as well as my right to sue the Released Parties.

________ (INITIALS)

OTHER MATTERS: I understand that the Released Parties make no representations, warranties or other promises, express or implied, regarding third party items provided at or during the course of the Activities (such as the safety of third party facilities or equipment and the like), even if those items are provided by, or at the recommendation of, the Released Parties. Similarly, the Released Parties may provide referrals to third parties who provide certain services related to the Activities (such as the names of gyms or fitness centers in the area), but make no representations, warranties or other promises, express or implied, regarding those services.

PUBLICITY RELEASE: I grant the Released Parties the right to photograph and/or videotape me and/or my child/ward and to use my and/or my child's/ward's name, face, likeness, voice and appearance in connection with exhibitions, publicity, advertising, and promotional materials without reservation or limitation.

I acknowledge that I have carefully read this release and waiver, and fully understand that it is a release of all liability and a waiver of any right that I may have on behalf of myself and/or my child/ward to bring a legal action or assert a claim for injury or loss of any kind against the released parties, even a claim based on the active or passive negligence of one or more of the released parties. If any attempt is made to make a claim, I understand I will be responsible for all defense costs incurred by the released parties.

If participant is under eighteen (18) years: I have read the above, been given the opportunity to ask questions, considered its effects, understand its content, and agree, on behalf of myself and my child/ward, to the terms as stated above. I warrant that I have full authority to agree and sign on behalf of my child/ward. I will further indemnify the Released Parties against any damages incurred as a result of any action by my child/ward including attorneys' fees and costs.

I have read the above, been given the opportunity to ask questions, considered its effects, understand its content, and agree, on behalf of myself and my child/ward, to the terms as stated above.

PRINTED NAME

SIGNATURE OF PARTICIPANT/PARENT/LEGAL GUARDIAN DATE

NAME OF CHILD PARTICIPANT BIRTH DATE

NAME OF CHILD PARTICIPANT BIRTH DATE

)(

The happiest excitement in life
is to be convinced that one is fighting
for all one is worth
on behalf of some clearly seen
and deeply felt good.

RUTH BENEDICT

)(

Action Items

The following list of action items can help the event organizers assign tasks, schedule timelines, establish deadlines, and monitor progress on a variety of fronts. The "point person" is the person who has lead responsibility for executing the assignment. Others may play secondary roles; indeed, coordination with one or more event organizers will be required for the execution of many tasks. Still, it is helpful to designate one lead person so that he or she is empowered to push the task to completion. Although the list suggests sequential actions, many of the tasks will overlap each other.

Before the First Session

Action	Point Person
Decide to create a Community Meltdown	Spokesperson
Select a chief executive officer (CEO)	Spokesperson
Establish a name for the event	Spokesperson and CEO
Issue a public challenge	Spokesperson and CEO
Recruit a core team of event organizers	Spokesperson and CEO
Distribute job descriptions and materials	CEO
Create a vision and establish goals	Core team members
Determine measurements for success	Core team members
Determine timing (number of sessions)	Core team members
Schedule dates for sessions	Core team members
Establish an office or work area	CEO
Develop a budget	CEO
Secure funding for necessary expenses	CEO
Establish a Web site and e-mail account	Media adviser
Establish a Web-based registration system	Registrar
Oversee distribution of registration forms	Registrar
Maintain a list of participants to talk to the media	Registrar
Seek endorsements	Core team members
Begin a promotional campaign	CEO and media adviser
Issue a public challenge	CEO, spokesperson, and media adviser
Identify existing communication networks	Media adviser
Create written material	Media adviser and spokesperson
Create a press kit	Media adviser
Create and distribute flyers and posters	Media adviser
Reserve a venue	Event producer
Obtain insurance for the event	Business and legal adviser
Draft policies and review written contracts	Business and legal adviser
Solicit prizes and awards	Prize and vendor coordinator
Write opening and closing procedures	Event producer and supervisor of volunteers
Coordinate event logistics	Event producer
Create directional and parking signs	Event producer and supervisor of volunteers
Make arrangements to offer special incentives	Fitness center liaison
Interview, select, and schedule presenters	Medical adviser

Plan special programs for the middle and final sessions	Spokesperson, CEO, and event producer
Arrange tie-ins with other fitness programs	Executive assistant to the CEO
Track expenses during the Community Meltdown	Executive assistant to the CEO
Order T-shirts and buttons to promote the event	Prize and vendor coordinator
Inventory prizes and donations; plan distribution	Prize and vendor coordinator
Assign and oversee volunteers for each session	Supervisor of volunteers

During the Sessions

Action	Point Person
Establish a team network and reporting system	Captain of captains
Broadcast e-mails to captains	Captain of captains
Manage media contacts	Media adviser
Stream information to the media	Media adviser
Update the Web site	Media adviser and webmaster
Establish a communication network for fitness centers	Fitness center liaison
Establish a communication network for volunteers	Supervisor of volunteers
Establish a team to produce the event	Event producer
Videotape sessions with clips for media coverage	Event producer and media adviser
Document all aspects of the event using various media and sources	Media adviser
Keep notes and records of the experience	Core team members
Set the tone for each session	Spokesperson

After the Last Session

Action	Point Person
Acknowledge and thank key players	Spokesperson, CEO, and core team members
Distribute participant evaluations	Webmaster or executive assistant to the CEO
Critique and celebrate results	Core team members
Write articles for the local media related to fitness	Spokesperson
Encourage participation in fitness programs	Spokesperson
Update the Web site and keep it fresh and new	CEO
Organize future fitness events	Core team members

)(

Before you begin a thing,
remind yourself that difficulties and delays
quite impossible to foresee are ahead.
If you could see them clearly,
naturally you could do a great deal
to get rid of them
but you can't.
You can only see one thing clearly
and that is your goal.
Form a mental vision of that
and cling to it through thick and thin.

KATHLEEN NORRIS

)(

Sample Team Registration Form

The team captain collects the information below for his or her team and forwards it to the registrar. This document officially registers the team and forms the basis for measuring progress and awarding prizes. The information is also used to communicate with participants as the need arises.

Team Registration Form

Team name		
Team captain	Phone	E-mail

	Member name	**Phone**	**E-mail**	**Starting weight**
1				
2				
3				
4				
5				
6				
7				
8				
	Number of members including captain		**Total team starting weight**	

Goals (may include goals other than weight; may include individual or collective goals):

Special interests:

Special needs/requests:

Signature of team captain:	**Date:**

Note: Use reverse side for additional members or for mailing addresses where e-mail addresses are unavailable.

Sample Team Formation Checklist

At the initial session and, to a lesser degree, at subsequent sessions, the event organizers will need to help strangers bond together and become a cohesive team. A facilitator can be assigned to each small group to help the individuals organize into a team. Facilitators can use this checklist to ensure that the essential elements of team formation are covered.

Team Formation Checklist

- ☐ *Exchange of information:* Do we all have each other's phone numbers and e-mail addresses and know how/when to get in touch?
- ☐ *Neighbors:* Do any of us live near each other? Could we take walks together?
- ☐ *Captain:* Who is our captain? Do we have the captain's phone number?
- ☐ *Weight:* What is the collective starting weight of the team?
- ☐ *Exercise:* What will be our exercise program?
- ☐ *Support:* What's the best way to support each other?
- ☐ *Reporting:* When will we send our weekly weight to the captain?
- ☐ *Goals:* What is our collective goal for the Community Meltdown? How many pounds do we want to lose?
- ☐ *Food diaries:* Will any of us keep food diaries or exchange tips?
- ☐ *Exercise dates:* Will we be exercising together? Do we want to organize walks?
- ☐ *Celebrations:* How will we celebrate little victories?
- ☐ *Weekly goals:* What is our goal for this week?

Roles and Responsibilities of Team Captains

Once a team has been formed, the teammates need to decide who will be captain. The list of tasks below can help the group decide who can comfortably take on the added responsibility.

Team Captains' Responsibilities

- *Exchange of information among teammates:* Make sure all participants have each other's phone numbers, e-mail addresses, or other ways to contact teammates.
- *Recordkeeping:* Keep the official team registration form, which includes individual starting weights and ending weights. Record progress each week.
- *Encouraging teammates to seek help:* Encourage team members to see their physician or an appropriate medical person before making lifestyle changes if the team members have medical concerns, limitations, injuries, or other conditions that require attention.
- *Exercise:* Encourage teammates to exercise and arrange exercise dates.
- *Food intake:* Encourage teammates to keep a diary of food intake.
- *Education:* Share any useful information with teammates.
- *Goal setting:* Encourage teammates to set and write down weekly goals. Record the goals for each person on the team.
- *Cheerleading:* Keep in contact with teammates and encourage them to continue their participation. Share good news and progress. Encourage teammates who may get discouraged.
- *Weekly reporting:* Report the results of the team (pounds lost) at each weekly session during roll call.
- *Final reporting:* Bring the final results to the final session. This includes starting team weight, final team weight, and the difference in weight.
- *Lightening up:* Have fun and a grand adventure yourself, and encourage your teammates to lighten up.

Roles and Responsibilities of Teammates

Teammates support each other and can make the team captain's job easier by staying in touch, responding to requests for information, and meeting deadlines for reporting information.

Teammates' Responsibilities

- *Exchange of information:* Collect and give information about how to contact each other.
- *Reporting:* Inform your team captain of your starting weight and progress week to week.
- *Seeking help:* See your physician or an appropriate medical person before making lifestyle changes if you have medical concerns, limitations, injuries, or other conditions that require attention.
- *Exercise:* Structure an exercise program appropriate for yourself and encourage your teammates to join you. Schedule exercise dates.
- *Food intake:* Keep a food diary. Note when you overeat and what triggers overeating.
- *Education:* Take every opportunity to educate yourself about exercise, nutrition, and health issues relating to fitness.
- *Goal setting:* Set personal goals. Communicate those goals to your captain.
- *Cheerleading:* Tell your family and friends about your goals. Ask for their support and encouragement. Encourage your teammates.
- *Weekly reporting:* Report your results to your captain before each weekly session.
- *Final reporting:* Report your final results to your captain before the final session.
- *Lightening up:* Have fun and a grand adventure, and encourage your teammates to do likewise.

Sample Weekly Reporting Form

Each week, captains need to report the results of their teams' efforts. To save time, a standard means of reporting the information needs to be developed. This sample form addresses that issue. The captain of captains needs to distribute this or a similar report form to all team captains to track their teams' weight losses over the sessions of the event.

Weekly Team Report

Team name		
Team captain	Phone	E-mail
Number of teammates	Overall ending weight goal	

	Group weight	Date
Session 1		
Session 2		
Session 3		
Session 4		
Session 5		
Session 6		
Session 7		
Session 8		

Summary	
Current week starting weight	
Current week ending weight	–
Difference	=

Sample Summary Statistical Reporting Form

The captain of captains collects information from the team captains and needs to standardize that information for ease of compilation and distribution. This or a similar report can be created as an Excel spreadsheet and used to tabulate the total weight-loss results. Color-coded tables are easier to read.

Team no.	Team name	Captain	Loss to date	Feb 16 team wt.	Week 6 loss	Loss to date	Feb 23 team wt.	Week 7 loss	Loss to date	Avg. loss per team
	Grass Valley United Methodist Church									
1	High Flyers	Fran Martin	-47	981	-9	-56	972	-9	-65	-11
2	Tons of Fun 1	Dee Norman	-43	922	0	-43	920	-2	-45	-8
3	We've Got Spirit	Dorothy Murray	-27	1125	-7	-34	1116	-9	-43	-6
4	Winsome Losers	Sandy Mangano	-35	1025	1	-34	1018	-7	-41	-7
201	Wild Women 2	Sheryl Slade	-12	778	-4	-16	0	0	-16	-4
202	Wildwood Bunch	Darlene Colman	-43	862	1	-42	856	-6	-48	-10
203	Winning Losers	Sunny Romalo	-39	955	-3	-42	949	-6	-48	-10
204	WOMBATS	Karlene Harter	-51	893	-5	-56	881	-12	-68	-14
205	Women on a Mission	Nan Berg	-5	1047	-25	-30	0	0	-30	-6
206	WWW Losers.com	Pam Stevens	-46	642	-2	-48	655	13	-35	-9
207	Yin Yang	Sue Diller	-25	920	-4	-29	898	-22	-51	-10
208	Z Dogs	Deb Paine	-8	898	-1	-9	0	0	-9	-2
			-5898	**189321**	**-696**	**-6594**	**178107**	**-910**	**-7504**	
			Total loss to date		**Week 6 loss**	**Total loss to date**		**Week 7 loss**	**Total loss to date**	

)(

We go where our vision is.

JOSEPH MURPHY

)(

Sample Community Fitness Resources List

We recommend that the event organizers pool their knowledge and compile a list of free or low-cost fitness opportunities in their community. Examples include hiking trails, public pools, tennis courts, parks, and running tracks. Free programs offered through parks, recreation departments, and other agencies, especially those oriented toward youth, need to be included.

Name	Description	Details	Location, hours, fee
Harrison Trail	0.6 mile to 2.1 miles	Easy	Take Harrison Road to College Drive. Park on street near entrance to paved walk. Free.
Union High School	Outdoor track	Easy	Union High School. Open to the public on weekends. Free.
Independence Trail	1.5 miles	Easy, handicapped accessible	Highway 49 north of Orion City. Free.
Union Park	2 outdoor tennis courts	Hard courts	Union Park in Orion City. Free.
Pascale Park	Outdoor lap pool	All ages	Pascale Park in Pascale. Open daily 8 AM–9 PM from June to August. Children ages 15 and under $0.75. Ages 16 and up, $1.25.
Centennial Park	4 outdoor tennis courts	Hard courts	Five miles southeast on McKee Highway in Orion City. Free.

Sample Fitness Club Internal Communication to Participants

Fitness center owners and trainers can encourage ongoing exercise activities by making sure new members feel welcome, educating members by offering helpful tips, pointing out unique opportunities, and conveying special promotional offers for membership. E-mails are an efficient yet personal way to stay in touch. A sample e-mail is presented below.

Subject: Tip for the Day

Go Meltdowners! We hope you are really benefiting from your time here at A Fitter You Athletic Club. Good job, everyone!

TIP FOR THE DAY!

Exercise may be more fun with a partner, but don't let lack of a partner keep you from exercising. When your partner calls in sick, be ready with a backup plan. Take a walk alone, or listen to a book on tape when you work out at a fitness center. If you like to be with people but lose your exercise partner, sign up for a group exercise class.

In case you don't already know, please ask any membership adviser about the Community Meltdown Membership Special that expires January 31.

Have a fun and fit day!

Materials to Bring to Each Session

The executive assistant to the CEO needs to bring, or arrange to be brought, materials for use by the event organizers at each session. This is a preliminary list of materials; other items can be added depending upon the content of the session. An asterisk indicates that a sample of this material is included in the appendix.

Materials for Sessions

- FAQs for Community Meltdown*
- Legal release for participants*
- Team registration form*
- Roles and responsibilities of team captains*
- Roles and responsibilities of teammates*
- Weekly reporting form*
- The ABCs of Fitness*
- Weekly prizes and awards
- Resource materials made available by health and wellness service providers (dietary guidelines, exercise options, signs of stroke, etc.)
- Paper, pens, and clipboards
- Fitness club passes
- Items to sell (buttons, Community Meltdown T-shirts, etc.)
- Weight scale
- Music (tapes, CDs, etc.)

* See sample in appendix.

Sample Postevent Evaluation Form

In order to evaluate the event, the event organizers need to decide which questions to ask and determine how responses will be measured. Information and instructions on how to complete an evaluation of the event can be e-mailed to participants by the captain of captains. The webmaster can also create an on-line evaluation form using several free survey services available on the Internet.

Postevent Evaluation Form

1. What was your team's name?	
2. What was your team's starting weight?	
3. How many pounds did your team lose?	
4. What was the age range on your team?	

5. Please check one response for each question below.

	0	1	2	3	4	5	6	7	8	9 or more
How many weeks has your team participated?										
How many women are on your team?										
How many men are on your team?										

6. Please check how frequently your team participated in the listed activities.

	Daily	3+ per week	1–2 per week	Less than 1 per week	At least 1 time	Never
E-mailed each other						
Attended weekly Community Meltdown session						
Exercised together at beginning of Community Meltdown						
Exercised together at end of Community Meltdown						
Exercised solo at beginning of Community Meltdown						
Exercised solo at end of Community Meltdown						
Used Community Meltdown Web site						
Shared health and fitness tips						
Socialized and had fun						

7. Please rank how important (1 = most important, 2 = 2nd most important, etc.) each of the following Community Meltdown elements was in your team's success.

	1	2	3	4	5	6	7	8
Being part of a team								
Gym passes								
Exercise regimen								

Changed eating habits								
Keeping food journal								
Changed shopping habits								
Information at Community Meltdown sessions								
Competing for prizes								

8. Please rank the importance (1 = most important, 2 = 2nd most important, etc.) of each of the following Community Meltdown outcomes for your team.

	1	2	3	4	5	6	7	8
Lost weight								
Healthier eating habits								
Improved fitness								
Identified sustainable life changes								
Made new friends/support system								
Strengthened existing support system								
Part of community event								
Understand fitness issues								

9. Would you participate in future Community Meltdown-type community initiatives?

Yes	
No	
Not sure	

10. What is the single most important success factor for you and your team?

11. How could the Community Meltdown or similar community initiatives be improved next time?

12. Please list your teammates and contact information (phone and e-mail) so we can contact them about their suggestions, as well as future events.

Index